Weight Watchers Air Fryer Cookbook 2021

Amazingly Easy and Delicious WW Smart Points Recipes to Fry, Bake, and Roast with Your Air Fryer

Alexa Trisler

Copyright© 2021 Alexa Trisler - All Rights Reserved.

In no way is it legal to reproduce, duplicate, or transmit any part of this document by either electronic means or in printed format. Recording of this publication is strictly prohibited, and any storage of this material is not allowed unless with written permission from the publisher. All rights reserved.

The information provided herein is stated to be truthful and consistent, in that any liability, regarding inattention or otherwise, by any usage or abuse of any policies, processes, or directions contained within is the solitary and complete responsibility of the recipient reader. Under no circumstances will any legal liability or blame be held against the publisher for any reparation, damages, or monetary loss due to the information herein, either directly or indirectly.

Respective authors own all copyrights not held by the publisher.

Legal Notice:

This book is copyright protected. This is only for personal use. You cannot amend, distribute, sell, use, quote or paraphrase any part of the content within this book without the consent of the author or copyright owner. Legal action will be pursued if this is breached.

Disclaimer Notice:

Please note the information contained within this document is for educational and entertainment purposes only. Every attempt has been made to provide accurate, up-to-date and reliable, complete information. No warranties of any kind are expressed or implied. Readers acknowledge that the author is not engaging in the rendering of legal, financial, medical or professional advice.

By reading this document, the reader agrees that under no circumstances are we responsible for any losses, direct or indirect, which are incurred as a result of the use of information contained within this document, including, but not limited to, errors, omissions, or inaccuracies.

Table of Content

Introduction 1
Chapter1: The Weight Watchers Basics 2
    The history of weight watchers 2
    What is SmartPoints? 2
    How do SmartPoints work? 3
    Freestyle pros and cons 4
    Food to eat 5
    Food to avoid 7
Chapter2: Success Tips for Weight Watchers Freestyle 8
Chapter3: FQAs 10
Chapter4: Breakfast 11
    Garlic Bread Bites 11
    Butternut Squash Falafel 12
    Turkey Bacon 14
    Grilled Cheese 15
    Breakfast Quiche 16
    Hard Boiled Eggs 18
    Pancakes 19
    Egg Scramble 20
Chapter5: Appetizer and Sides 21
    Butternut Squash Fries 21
    Plantain 22
    Asparagus 23
    Pizza 24
    Fried Pickle Chips 25
    Spiced Chickpeas 26
    Corn on Cob 27
    Shishito Peppers 28
Chapter6: Beef, Lamb, and Pork 29

Short Ribs 29

Meatloaf 30

Lamb Chops 32

Roast Beef 33

Empanadas 34

Herb Crusted Pork Chops 36

Pork Taquitos 37

Breaded Pork Chops 38

Honey Mustard Pork Chops 40

Steak 41

Meatballs 42

Lamb Chops 43

Chapter7: Poultry 44

Chicken Parmesan 44

Buffalo Chicken Taquitos 45

Feta Stuffed Chicken 45

Chicken Shawarma Salad 47

Turkey Breast 49

Chicken Nuggets 50

Cheesy Ranch Chicken 51

Whole Roasted Chicken 52

Chapter8: Vegetarian 54

Vegetable Kebab 55

Baked Potatoes 56

Savory Squash Wedges 57

Cajun Zucchini Chips 58

Buffalo Cauliflower Wings 59

Brussels Sprouts 60

Green Beans 61

Chapter9: Fish and Seafood 62

Salt and Pepper Shrimp 62

Tuna Cakes 63

Coconut Shrimp 64

Ranch Fish Fillets 65

Fried Cat Fish 66

Sriracha Salmon 67

Fish Sticks 68

Cilantro Lime Shrimp Skewers 70

Salmon Patties 72

Chapter10: Desserts 73

Pop Tarts 73

Apple Chips with Cinnamon 74

Lemon Muffins 75

Pumpkin Spiced Cookies 76

Carrot Cake 78

Funnel Cake Bites 79

Cinnamon Rolls 81

Conclusion 82

Introduction

Everyone loves food; it makes us healthy and happy. And, this means everyone should eat everything. Then what about those diets that stop you from eating certain foods? Obviously, these diets have a strong reason to emphasize healthy eating habits that keeps the body strong and fit and most importantly, maintain their body shape.

How about I tell you that there is a healthy lifestyle that doesn't believe in telling you what you eat or not. This diet doesn't believe that any food should be forbidden. This diet is called the Weight Watchers Freestyle. Weight Watchers Freestyle is science-based food management that provides information, tools and community that educates you to make a right healthy eating decision and about exercise. Moreover, it also Weight Watchers Freestyle also encourage you to enjoy what you eat. And the best part, Weight Watchers Freestyle has immensely gained success in personal weight loss compared to other weight loss program.

It is all about Weight Watchers knowledge and your efforts that bring positive behavioral changes and inspire and motivate you in every step to lose weight and leading a healthy life.

Chapter1: The Weight Watchers Basics

The history of weight watchers

So, the story of Weight Watchers is built around a simple philosophy of around empathy, mutual understanding, and rapport. It began in September 1061 when Jean, an overweight woman from Queens, New York, found her motivation waning by just losing 20 pounds of weight by sticking to a popular fad diet promoted by New York City Board of Health. She had spent a year in the desperation of losing weight, but the result wasn't fruitful. In her misery, her few overweight friends and confessed about her obsession with food. Her friends not only understood her addiction to food, but they also shared their food obsessions too and decided to meet each other every week for mutual support and sharing their overwhelming journey of losing weight. And, the word spread about this support group and more people became part of Jean caring group, they soon realized that controlling weight wasn't just about dieting, it is much more than that.

Along with eating healthy food, losing weight also require a change in habits and continuous support and encouragement from family, friend, and people who cared. The realization of healthy lifestyle management through empathy and sharing led Jean to lose 70 pounds weight and resulted in the formation of one of the most successful scientific weight management organization in 1963. Even today, Weight Watchers promote physical, emotional and mental health.

What is SmartPoints?

Eating on Weight Watchers is based on SmartPoints. SmartPoints gives the value of what you are consuming as food. SmartPoints is basically a counting system that uses a counting system with the help of nutritional science. The reason this nutritional value system is called smart because it motivates to eat healthy and nutritious food so that you feel better, live better, keep energy level highs throughout the day and lose weight. Here's how SmartPoints works:

- SmartPoints are given to a food based on its calories, protein, sugar and saturated fats. Calories are the baseline of SmartPoints; protein lowers the value of smart points whereas fat and sugar increase points.
- You can set your goals according to your food or drink plans and keep track of your points as you consume the food.
- Even if your weekend meal differs from the rest of the week, you can roll over your SmartPoints automatically whenever you want. Rollovers add flexibility to use SmartPoints to roll over unused points when you need them in any day like for special occasions, weekends, a second helping and much more.
- And the best of all, there are more than 200 foods that have zero SmartPoints. Therefore, you don't have to track or measure SmartPoints. These foods include chicken breast, turkey breast, salmon, shrimps, oysters, shellfish, beans, lentils, tofu, nonfat yogurt and vegetables including peas and corn, etc.

How do SmartPoints work?

You can set your daily and weekly SmartPoints. So, here's how you can set your target.

SmartPoints target on a daily basis is set according to age, gender, height, and weight and these factors help in calculating that you get sufficient nutrients and energy to perform important activities throughout the day and also, lost weight. Similarly, you can use your daily SmartPoints to set your weekly SmartPoints target.

You can also track your weekly SmartPoints target using Weight Watchers app at https://www.weightwatchers.com/uk/weight-watchers-app to sort out the rest. Not only it tracks your food and drinks, but the app also monitors quickly monitor and view your weight and activity progress. You can also browse through foods and recipes and even restaurants. Last but not least, you share your weight loss victories on the platform and even can get instant advice from an online coach.

Freestyle pros and cons

Following are some fantastic benefits and drawbacks of Weight Watchers Freestyle. These list of pros and cons can decide if Weight Watchers Freestyle is right for you or not.

Pros:

- Unlimited Choices: You can eat anything you want as long as you can track its SmartPoints.
- Promote Whole Foods: The lowest points of food on Weight Watchers Freestyle is zero that can be acquired from protein sources like meat, seafood and yogurt and vegetables, and fruits.
- Teaches You to Make Better Lifestyle Choices: By tracking the SmartPoints using calories, nutrients and its effect on weight, Weight Watchers Freestyle teach dieters to allow them to decide whether the food they are having worth the points.
- Support: Weight Watchers Freestyle offers support 24/7 through weekly meetings, discussions, and weigh-ins.
- Community: Weight Watchers Freestyle has a massive community of people who understand what you are going through and are there to give you valuable nutritional tips, share information, cooking advice, their food experiences that help you achieve your health goals.
- Achieve Steady Weight Loss: You can expect to lose up to two pounds of weight every week on Weight Watchers Freestyle program. You can even lose more in the start but remember, weight loss is a steady process, and your goal should be consistently losing weight.
- Promote Exercise: Weight Watchers Freestyle program encourages indulging into physical activities. The physical movement gives your Fitpoints that you can use to balance your food intake. You can begin with light exercise and then move on to work harder to burn more calories.

- Encourage Home Cooking: The secret of healthy cooking relates to cooking fresh food by yourself. Weight Watchers Freestyle program offers thousands of easy and tasty recipes that will help you proficient in preparing food that will keep your body lean, strong and fit.

Cons:

- It Is Expensive: There is a fee for the online program. The plan starts with $4.61 per week. But the monetary investment in the program depends on the level you are choosing. The membership fee is minimal and significant if you have to lose lots of weight. Just be sure you calculate the entire cost of your plan and make sure you can afford it.
- Weekly weigh-in of the body is necessary: You need to weigh in to track your progress. For some dieters, this requirement helps dieters to keep on track on this program, while for some, it is uncomfortable. If you are following the program to the T and doing it the right way, then you will steadily lose weight.
- Counting SmartPoints is Tedious: If you don't like counting, then you may not like counting for tracking SmartPoints. Counting SmartPoints can sometimes be a time-consuming and complicated task, especially for those dieters who are seeking something quick and straightforward approach of a healthy lifestyle.

Food to eat

You need to pay attention to eat those foods that have fewer points on the Weight Watchers program. The following food list will help you meet your SmartPoints target:

Meat:

- Skinless chicken breast
- Chicken thighs (boneless)
- Turkey breast
- Beef and steaks

- Turkey bacon
- Ham
- Pork Chops
- Fish
- Seafood

Vegetables:

- Tomatoes, mixed salad greens, green beans, carrots, sweet potato, sweet red peppers, mushrooms, potato (white or red), grape tomato
- Corn on Cob

Fruits:

- Banana, apple, strawberries, blueberries, raspberries, grapes, watermelon, avocado, lettuce, pineapple, peach, pears

Grains, Beans, Rice

- Bread
- English Muffin
- Hamburger bun
- Bagel
- Tortillas
- Beans
- Peas
- Oatmeal
- White rice and brown rice
- Quinoa
- Almonds

Fats:

- Olive oil
- Butter
- Peanut butter

Poultry:

- Eggs
- Yogurt (nonfat)
- Coffee (unsweetened)
- Diet Coke
- White wine and red wine
- Milk (fat-free) including almond milk
- Half-and-half
- Cheddar cheese, American cheese, Parmesan cheese, cottage cheese, feta cheese
- Greek Yogurt (nonfat)

Condiments:

- Salsa
- Hummus
- Mustard
- Salad dressing
- Guacamole

Food to avoid

No food is forbidden on Weight Watchers Freestyle. However, the following are some foods that you should limit.

- Fast food
- Hamburger
- Pizza
- Cake
- Ice cream (sweetened)
- Soda

Chapter2: Success Tips for Weight Watchers Freestyle

- Stay Hydrated: Keeping your hydrated during Weight Watchers Freestyle program is very important, whether you are aiming for weight loss or not. Make sure you have at least one water bottle, about 500 mL, with you every time. Sip it throughout the day and make an objective to drink four water bottles during the day as this will supply eight glasses of water per day. Don't worry if you don't meet this objective at the beginning of this program. Just concentrate on drinking more, the more you drink, the more easily you will drink all four bottles down. You can also add stevia to improve the taste of water or have lemonade in place of it.
- Eat Fresh Veggies and Fruits: Fruits and vegetables have zero SmartPoints on Weight Watchers Freestyle. The minute you buy them, wash and cut them up and store so that you can enjoy them at any time of the day.
- Variety: Since you can eat anything on Weight Watchers Freestyle, so make sure you eat different foods throughout the day. Add variety in your meals. Even better, make a list of your favorite food and have them ready beforehand like boiled eggs, pre-cooked chicken and so on. In this way, you knew what you are looking forward to eating that will fill and satisfy your stomach.
- No Unnecessary Work: You don't have to work unnecessary for Weight Watchers Freestyle. Although, Weight Watchers Freestyle promote harvesting your own veggies and fruits, but it sounds like work, don't go for it. Yes, that's actually one of the benefits of flexible Weight Watchers Freestyle that it can accommodate to any lifestyle.
- Use Air Fryer: Just because you have healthy eating food, that doesn't mean that you have to forbid yourself having fried foods. Yes, you can enjoy that crispiness of fried food on Weight Watchers Freestyle by using an air fryer. An air fryer is a great appliance when you want to eat oil-

less healthy and crunchy food. Our air fryer recipes in chapter 4 for Weight Watchers Freestyle is a great place to start.

Chapter3: FQAs

Question: Is this program like Keto?

Answer: No, Ketogenic diet is a restrictive diet that allows only high-fat, protein-rich and very low carb foods. On the other hand, Weight Watchers Freestyle has everything on their menu and dieters can choose to eat anything freely.

Question: What are ZeroPoint foods?

Answer: ZeroPoint foods are made up of protein, vegetables, fruits, and saturated fats. These foods contain high nutrition and provide a foundation of healthy eating patterns without posing any risk of health in case of overeating.

Question: Which foods included in the list of zero SmartPoints?

Answer: Skinless chicken and turkey breast including thighs, ground chicken, deli meat, turkey bacon, fish, seafood, eggs, yogurt, cheese, beans, peas, corn, lentil, vegetables, and fruits.

Question: Why meats like beef, lamb, and pork are not part of ZeroPoint foods like a chicken breast on Weight Watchers Freestyle?

Answer: Beef, lamb, and pork are recommended to consume every week under limits on Weight Watchers Freestyle as the overconsumption of these foods increase the risks for cancer and coronary ailment. However, on Weight Watchers Freestyle you can enjoy meats using your SmartPoints budgets.

Question: Beans and peas are high in carbs so what do they have zero SmartPoints?

Answer: Beans and peas and other variety of high carb and starchy vegetables, fruits, lentils, and legumes are naturally high in fiber compare to other foods. Also, they are filling and nutritious, and that's why they are encouraged to eat more on Weight Watchers Freestyle.

Chapter4: Breakfast

Garlic Bread Bites

Servings: 8
Total time: 20 minutes

Nutrition Value:

Calories: 160 Cal, Carbs: 18.7 g, Fat: 7.5 g, Protein: 3.5 g, Fiber: 1.3 g.

Smart Points Per Serving: 3

Ingredients:

- 1 cup self-rising flour, divided
- ½ teaspoon garlic salt
- ½ teaspoon dried parsley
- 1 cup Greek yogurt, nonfat

Method:

1. Place ¾ cup flour in a bowl, add garlic salt, parsley and yogurt and stir until mixed.
2. Transfer dough onto a clean working space, sprinkle with flour, roll and then cut into 32 squares.
3. Switch on the air fryer, then insert fryer basket greased with non-stick cooking spray, shut with its lid and preheat at 375 degrees F for 5 minutes.
4. Open air fryer, place squares into the pan in a single layer, then shut with lid and cook at 325 degrees F for 10 minutes, flipping bites halfway through.
5. When air fryer beeps, open the air fryer, transfer garlic bites to a plate and serve.

Butternut Squash Falafel

Servings: 2

Total time: 40 minutes

Nutrition Value:

Calories: 182 Cal, Carbs: 36 g, Fat: 2 g, Protein: 7 g, Fiber: 8 g.

Smart Points Per Serving: 0

Ingredients:

- 14-ounce cooked chickpeas
- 10-ounce butternut squash, peeled and cubed
- ½ of white onion, peeled and chopped
- ½ teaspoon minced garlic
- 1/2 teaspoon sea salt
- 1/8 teaspoon cayenne pepper
- 1 teaspoon ground cumin
- 1 teaspoon ground coriander
- 3 tablespoons chopped cilantro

Method:

1. Switch on the air fryer, then insert fryer basket greased with non-stick cooking spray, shut with its lid and preheat at 425 degrees F for 5 minutes.
2. Then add butternut squash pieces, spray with oil and shut with lid.
3. Cook butternut squash for 15 minutes until tender, shaking the basket halfway through.
4. When air fryer beeps, open the air fryer, transfer butternut squash into a food processor and add remaining ingredients.
5. Pulse for 2 to 3 minutes or until combined, then shape into balls and spray with cooking oil.

6. Place falafel balls into air fryer in a single layer, shut with lid and cook for 10 to 15 minutes or until nicely golden brown.
7. Serve straightaway.

Turkey Bacon

Servings: 8

Total time: 20 minutes

Nutrition Value:

Calories: 30 Cal, Carbs: 0 g, Fat: 1.5 g, Protein: 6 g, Fiber: 0 g.

Smart Points Per Serving: 1

Ingredients:

- 8-ounce turkey bacon, uncured

Method:

1. Switch on the air fryer, then insert fryer basket greased with non-stick cooking spray, shut with its lid and preheat at 360 degrees F for 5 minutes.
2. Meanwhile, slice bacon into half.
3. Open air fryer, place bacon halves into heated fryer basket, then shut with lid and cook at 325 degrees F for 10 minutes, turning bacon halfway through.
4. When air fryer beeps, open the air fryer, transfer bacon to plates.
5. Serve straightaway.

Grilled Cheese

Servings: 8

Total time: 20 minutes

Nutrition Value:

Calories: 366 Cal, Carbs: 28 g, Fat: 23 g, Protein: 12 g, Fiber: 1.4 g.

Smart Points Per Serving: 3

Ingredients:

- 2 slices of bread
- 1 slice of Velveeta cheese

Method:

1. Switch on the air fryer, then insert fryer basket greased with non-stick cooking spray, shut with its lid and preheat at 350 degrees F for 5 minutes.
2. Meanwhile, sandwich cheese slice between bread slices and spray with oil
3. Open air fryer, place the sandwich into heated fryer basket, then shut with lid and cook for 8 minutes, flipping sandwich halfway through.
4. When air fryer beeps, open the air fryer, transfer sandwich to a cutting board and cut in half.
5. Serve straightaway.

Breakfast Quiche

Servings: 8
Total time: 35 minutes

Nutrition Value:

Calories: 151.8 Cal, Carbs: 3.6 g, Fat: 10.2 g, Protein: 11.3 g, Fiber: 0.4 g.

Smart Points Per Serving: 4

Ingredients:

- ½ cup shredded mozzarella cheese
- 2/3 cup asparagus
- ¾ teaspoon salt
- ½ teaspoon ground black pepper
- 5 cherry tomatoes, quartered
- ⅓ cup diced green bell pepper
- 3 eggs
- 4 egg whites

Method:

1. Switch on the air fryer, then insert fryer proof pan greased with non-stick cooking spray, shut with its lid and preheat at 350 degrees F for 10 minutes.
2. Meanwhile, crack eggs and egg whites in a bowl, season with salt and black pepper and whisk until beaten.
3. Cut asparagus into 1-inch pieces, add to eggs along with pepper, and tomatoes, stir until combined, then add half of the cheese and stir until mixed.
4. Open air fryer, spoon quiche mixture into fryer pan, then shut with lid and cook for 20 minutes or until quiche is set and the top is nicely golden brown.

5. When air fryer beeps, open the air fryer, remove the pan from air fryer and take out quiche.
6. Let quiche cool for 5 minutes and then slice to serve.

Hard Boiled Eggs

Servings: 2

Total time: 30 minutes

Nutrition Value:

Calories: 78 Cal, Carbs: 0.5 g, Fat: 5.3 g, Protein: 6.3 g, Fiber: 0 g.

Smart Points Per Serving: 0

Ingredients:

- 4 eggs

Method:

1. Switch on the air fryer, then insert fryer basket, shut with its lid and preheat at 250 degrees F for 10 minutes.
2. Then open the air fryer, insert a wire rack, place eggs on it, shut with lid and cook for 16 minutes.
3. When air fryer beeps, open the air fryer and transfer eggs into a large bowl containing ice water to cool eggs.
4. When eggs are cooled, peel them and slice to serve.

Pancakes

Servings: 1

Total time: 11 minutes

Nutrition Value:

Calories: 78 Cal, Carbs: 10 g, Fat: 3.5 g, Protein: 1.8 g, Fiber: 0.5 g.

Smart Points Per Serving: 0

Ingredients:

- 1 medium banana, peeled
- 1/8 teaspoon ground cinnamon
- 1/16 teaspoon baking powder
- ½ teaspoon vanilla extract, unsweetened
- 2 eggs

Method:

1. Switch on the air fryer, then insert air fryer proof pan greased with non-stick cooking spray, shut with its lid and preheat at 220 degrees F for 5 minutes.
2. Meanwhile, place the banana in a medium bowl, mash with a fork, then add cinnamon, baking powder, vanilla and eggs and whisk until combined.
3. Open air fryer, pour prepared pancake batter in portions and spread it.
4. Then shut with lid and cook at 220 degrees F for 3 minutes, then flip the pancakes and continue cooking for another 3 minutes.
5. When air fryer beeps, open the air fryer, transfer pancakes to a plate and serve.

Egg Scramble

Servings: 10

Total time: 20 minutes

Nutrition Value:

Calories: 91 Cal, Carbs: 1 g, Fat: 6.7 g, Protein: 6.1 g, Fiber: 0 g.

Smart Points Per Serving: 3

Ingredients:

- 1/2 tomato, diced
- 2 cups baby spinach
- ½ of medium red onion, peeled and diced
- ¼ teaspoon minced garlic
- ¾ teaspoon salt
- ¾ teaspoon ground black pepper
- 6 tablespoons grated cheddar cheese
- 1 tablespoon olive oil
- 4 eggs

Method:

1. Switch on the air fryer, then insert fryer proof pan grease, add oil, shut with its lid and preheat at 220 degrees F for 1 minute.
2. Then add tomato, spinach, onion, and garlic, shut with lid and cook for 5 minutes until vegetables to tender.
3. Meanwhile, crack eggs in a bowl, add salt, black pepper and whisk until beaten.
4. Add whisked eggs into fryer pan, stir well, shut with lid and cook for 2 minutes.
5. Then stir eggs and continue cooking for 2 minutes.
6. When air fryer beeps, open the air fryer, transfer eggs into a plate, top with cheese and serve.

Chapter 5: Appetizer and Sides

Butternut Squash Fries

Servings: 8

Total time: 15 minutes

Nutrition Value:

Calories: 112.7 Cal, Carbs: 13.9 g, Fat: 6.9 g, Protein: 1.2 g, Fiber: 3.9 g.

Smart Points Per Serving: 0

Ingredients:

- 1-pound butternut squash
- 1 teaspoon salt
- ½ teaspoon red chili powder

Method:

1. Switch on the air fryer, then insert fryer basket greased with non-stick cooking spray, shut with its lid and preheat at 400 degrees F for 5 minutes.
2. Meanwhile, peel butternut squash, then remove its seeds and cut into ¾-inch long wedges.
3. Place butternut squash fries into a bowl, add salt and red chili powder and toss until coated.
4. Open air fryer, place fries into heated fryer basket, then shut with lid and cook for 8 minutes, shaking the basket every 2 minutes.
5. Serve straightaway.

Plantain

Servings: 2

Total time: 25 minutes

Nutrition Value:

Calories: 102 Cal, Carbs: 27 g, Fat: 0 g, Protein: 1 g, Fiber: 2 g.

Smart Points Per Serving: 5

Ingredients:

- 6-ounce green plantain, ends trimmed
- 3/4 teaspoon garlic powder
- 1 teaspoon salt
- 1 cup water

Method:

1. Switch on the air fryer, then insert fryer basket greased with non-stick cooking spray, shut with its lid and preheat at 400 degrees F for 5 minutes.
2. Meanwhile, peel plantain and cut into 1-inch thick slices.
3. Open air fryer, place plantain into heated fryer basket in a single layer, spray with oil, then shut with lid and cook for 6 minutes, shaking the basket halfway through.
4. When air fryer beeps, open the air fryer, transfer plantain to a plate and air fry remaining plantains in the same manner.
5. Pour water in a bowl, add garlic powder and salt and stir until salt is dissolved completely.
6. Mash plantain with a cup or bottom of a jar, then dip them into salty water and set aside.
7. Return these plantains into the air fryer, spray with oil and cook for 10 minutes, flipping halfway through.
8. When done, season plantains with more salt and serve.

Asparagus

Servings: 7

Total time: 20 minutes

Nutrition Value:

Calories: 45 Cal, Carbs: 3.9 g, Fat: 3 g, Protein: 2.2 g, Fiber: 1.9 g.

Smart Points Per Serving: 0

Ingredients:

- ½ bunch of asparagus
- 1 teaspoon salt

Method:

1. Switch on the air fryer, then insert fryer basket greased with non-stick cooking spray, shut with its lid and preheat at 400 degrees F for 5 minutes.
2. Meanwhile, trim the ends of asparagus, spray with oil and season with salt.
3. Open air fryer, place asparagus in a single layer into heated fryer basket, then shut with lid and cook for 8 minutes, shaking the basket halfway through.
4. When air fryer beeps, open the air fryer, transfer asparagus to a plate.
5. Serve straightaway.

Pizza

Servings: 4

Total time: 25 minutes

Nutrition Value:

Calories: 280 Cal, Carbs: 27 g, Fat: 14 g, Protein: 11 g, Fiber: 3 g.

Smart Points Per Serving: 3

Ingredients:

- 1 cup self-rising flour
- 4 slices of turkey pepperoni
- ½ teaspoon salt
- ½ teaspoon ground black pepper
- ½ teaspoon garlic powder
- 3 tablespoons pizza sauce
- 1 cup greek yogurt, non-fat
- 3 tablespoons grated cheddar cheese

Method:

1. Switch on the air fryer, then insert fryer basket greased with non-stick cooking spray, shut with its lid and preheat at 400 degrees F for 10 minutes.
2. Meanwhile, place flour in a bowl, add yogurt and stir until well mixed.
3. Transfer dough to a clean working space, then roll into crust and cut into 4 pieces.
4. Open air fryer, place crust pieces into heated fryer basket, then shut with lid and cook for 5 minutes.
5. Then transfer crust to a clean working space, spread sauce on top, add pepperoni slices and top with cheese.
6. Return pizza into the air fryer and cook for 7 to 10 minutes or until cooked through.
7. Serve straightaway.

Fried Pickle Chips

Servings: 6

Total time: 18 minutes

Nutrition Value:

Calories: 59 Cal, Carbs: 11.5 g, Fat: 0.5 g, Protein: 2.5 g, Fiber: 2 g.

Smart Points Per Serving: 2

Ingredients:

- 24 dill pickle chips
- 1/4 teaspoon onion powder
- 1/4 teaspoon garlic powder
- 1/4 teaspoon salt
- 1/4 teaspoon ground black pepper
- 1/8 teaspoon cayenne pepper
- 1/3 cup whole-wheat panko breadcrumbs
- 2 egg whites

Method:

1. Switch on the air fryer, then insert fryer basket greased with non-stick cooking spray, shut with its lid and preheat at 400 degrees F for 10 minutes.
2. Meanwhile, place breadcrumbs in a bowl, add onion powder, garlic powder, salt, black pepper, and cayenne pepper and stir until mixed.
3. Crack eggs in another bowl and whisk until blended.
4. Working on one pickle at a time, first dredge into the egg mixture and then coat with breadcrumbs mixture.
5. Open air fryer, place pickles in a single layer into heated fryer basket, spray with oil, then shut with lid and cook for 8 minutes, flipping pickles halfway through.
6. Cook remaining pickles in the same manner and serve.

7.
Spiced Chickpeas

Servings: 2

Total time: 20 minutes

Nutrition Value:

Calories: 187.1 Cal, Carbs: 24.2 g, Fat: 7.4 g, Protein: 7.3 g, Fiber: 6.3 g.

Smart Points Per Serving: 0

Ingredients:

- 16-ounce cooked chickpeas
- 1/2 teaspoon salt
- 1 teaspoon smoked paprika
- 1/8 teaspoon cayenne pepper
- 1/2 teaspoon ground cumin
- 1/2 tablespoon olive oil

Method:

1. Switch on the air fryer, then insert fryer basket greased with non-stick cooking spray, shut with its lid and preheat at 390 degrees F for 5 minutes.
2. Meanwhile, place chickpeas in a bowl, add remaining ingredients and stir well until chickpeas are coated with spices.
3. Open air fryer, add chickpeas into heated fryer basket, then shut with lid and cook for 15 minutes, shaking the basket halfway through.
4. When air fryer beeps, open the air fryer, transfer chickpeas to a bowl, let cool for 10 minutes and serve.

Corn on Cob

Servings: 3

Total time: 20 minutes

Nutrition Value:

Calories: 58 Cal, Carbs: 14.1 g, Fat: 0.5 g, Protein: 2 g, Fiber: 1.8 g.

Smart Points Per Serving: 0

Ingredients:

- 3 corn on the cobs
- 1 teaspoon salt
- Chopped cilantro for garnishing

Method:

1. Switch on the air fryer, then insert fryer basket greased with non-stick cooking spray, shut with its lid and preheat at 400 degrees F for 10 minutes.
2. Meanwhile, spray corns with oil and season with salt.
3. Open air fryer, place seasoned corns into heated fryer basket, then shut with lid and cook for 10 minutes, turning every 3 minutes.
4. When air fryer beeps, open the air fryer, transfer corn on the cob to a plate, sprinkle with cilantro and serve.

Shishito Peppers

Servings: 2

Total time: 20 minutes

Nutrition Value:

Calories: 21 Cal, Carbs: 5 g, Fat: 27 g, Protein: 6 g, Fiber: 2 g.

Smart Points Per Serving: 0

Ingredients:

- 20 shishito peppers
- ¾ teaspoon salt

Method:

1. Switch on the air fryer, then insert fryer basket greased with non-stick cooking spray, shut with its lid and preheat at 390 degrees F for 10 minutes.
2. Meanwhile, spray peppers with oil and season with salt.
3. Open air fryer, place seasoned peppers into heated fryer basket, then shut with lid and cook for 6 minutes or until lightly charred, shaking the basket halfway through.
4. When air fryer beeps, open the air fryer, transfer peppers to a plate.
5. Serve straightaway.

Chapter 6: Beef, Lamb, and Pork

Short Ribs

Servings: 8
Total time: 20 minutes

Nutrition Value:

Calories: 105 Cal, Carbs: 0 g, Fat: 6 g, Protein: 10 g, Fiber: 0 g.

Smart Points Per Serving: 1

Ingredients:

- 4 pounds short ribs
- 1/3 cup chopped green onion
- 1 tablespoon grated ginger
- 1 teaspoon ground black pepper
- 1/8 cup brown sugar
- 1 cup soy sauce
- 1 tablespoon sriracha sauce
- ½ cup rice vinegar

Method:

1. Stir together all the ingredients except for ribs in a bowl, stir until mixed and place in a large plastic bowl.
2. Ad short ribs into the bag, seal it and then turn it upside down until ribs are coated with prepared sauce.
3. Place the plastic bag in the refrigerator and let marinate for 4 hours or overnight.
4. When ready to cook, switch on the air fryer, then insert fryer basket greased with non-stick cooking spray, shut with its lid and preheat at 380 degrees F for 10 minutes.
5. Open air fryer, place ribs in a single layer into heated fryer basket, then shut with lid and cook for 8 minutes, flipping ribs halfway through.
6. Serve straightaway.

Meatloaf

Servings: 8

Total time: 35 minutes

Nutrition Value:

Calories: 457 Cal, Carbs: 20 g, Fat: 29 g, Protein: 26 g, Fiber: 1 g.

Smart Points Per Serving: 10

Ingredients:

- 1.5-pound ground beef
- 4 tablespoons chopped chorizo
- 1 medium green bell pepper, deseeded and grated
- 1 small white onion, peeled and grated
- 3/4 cup breadcrumbs
- 1 ½ teaspoon Salt
- ¾ teaspoon ground Black pepper
- 1 ½ tablespoon brown sugar
- 1 tablespoon and 1 teaspoon Dijon mustard paste
- 1 tablespoon Worcestershire sauce
- 3 tablespoons grated Parmesan cheese
- 1 tablespoon apple cider vinegar
- 2 eggs
- 7 tablespoons ketchup, divided

Method:

1. Switch on the air fryer, then insert fryer basket greased with non-stick cooking spray, shut with its lid and preheat at 390 degrees F for 10 minutes.
2. Meanwhile, place ground beef in a large bowl, add chorizo and rest of the ingredients except for brown sugar, vinegar, 1 teaspoon mustard and 4 tablespoon ketchup.

3. Stir well and shape the beef mixture into a meatloaf in an aluminum foil.
4. Open air fryer, place meatloaf into heated fryer basket, then shut with lid and cook for 20 to 30 minutes, shaking the basket halfway through.
5. In the meantime, prepare glaze for meatloaf by whisking together sugar, vinegar, mustard, and ketchup until blended.
6. When air fryer beeps, open the air fryer, brush prepare glaze on top and air fryer for another 5 minutes.
7. When done, transfer meatloaf to a cutting board, let stand for 10 minutes and then serve.

Lamb Chops

Servings: 4

Total time: 22 minutes

Nutrition Value:

Calories: 214 Cal, Carbs: 1.1 g, Fat: 12.4 g, Protein: 23.4 g, Fiber: 0.1 g.

Smart Points Per Serving: 3

Ingredients:

- 8 lamb chops
- 1 bulb of garlic
- 1 teaspoon sea salt
- ¾ teaspoon ground black pepper
- 1 tablespoon chopped oregano
- 3 tablespoons olive oil

Method:

1. Switch on the air fryer, then insert fryer basket greased with non-stick cooking spray, shut with its lid and preheat at 400 degrees F for 5 minutes.
2. Meanwhile, coat garlic bulb with oil.
3. Open air fryer, place garlic into heated fryer basket, then shut with lid and cook for 12 minutes.
4. Meanwhile, stir together remaining ingredients in a bowl until mixed, then coat ½ tablespoon of this mixture on lamb chops and marinate for 5 minutes.
5. When air fryer beeps, open the air fryer, transfer garlic bulb to a bowl and set aside.
6. Add marinated lamb chops into the air fryer basket, shut with lid and cook for 5 minutes or until nicely golden brown.
7. Squeeze garlic from their bulb, add to herbed oil and stir until well mixed.
8. Serve lamb chops with garlic herb sauce.

Roast Beef

Servings: 6

Total time: 1 hour

Nutrition Value:

Calories: 293 Cal, Carbs: 6 g, Fat: 27 g, Protein: 6 g, Fiber: 0 g.

Smart Points Per Serving: 3

Ingredients:

- 2-pound beef chuck roast, fat trimmed
- 1 teaspoon salt
- 1 teaspoon rosemary
- 1 tablespoon olive oil

Method:

1. Switch on the air fryer, then insert fryer basket greased with non-stick cooking spray, shut with its lid and preheat at 360 degrees F for 5 minutes.
2. Meanwhile, stir together salt, rosemary, and oil in a shallow dish, then add beef and turn it until well coated with the salt-rosemary mixture.
3. Open air fryer, place beef roast into heated fryer basket, then shut with lid and cook for 45 minutes or until cooked to desired doneness, turning beef halfway through.
4. When air fryer beeps, open the air fryer, transfer beef to a cutting board, then wrap with aluminum foil and let rest for 10 minutes.
5. Cut beef against the grain and serve.

Empanadas

Servings: 4

Total time: 30 minutes

Nutrition Value:

Calories: 207 Cal, Carbs: 18 g, Fat: 12 g, Protein: 6.7 g, Fiber: 0.9 g.

Smart Points Per Serving: 3

Ingredients:

- 1 cup self-rising flour, divided
- 1 cup cooked minced chicken
- ½ cup corn
- 2 teaspoons garlic powder
- ½ teaspoon salt
- ¼ cup tomato salsa
- 1 cup Greek yogurt, nonfat
- 1 egg, beaten

Method:

1. Switch on the air fryer, then insert fryer basket greased with non-stick cooking spray, shut with its lid and preheat at 325 degrees F for 10 minutes.
2. Meanwhile, place ¾ cup flour in a bowl, add yogurt and garlic powder and stir until well combined.
3. Transfer the dough on a clean working space, sprinkle with remaining dough, roll it out, divide evenly into 4 pieces and roll it out thinly.
4. Fill half of each dough pieces with chicken, then season with salsa, top with corn and salsa, fold over the remaining dough.
5. Seal the edges of empanadas by pressing the edges with fork and brush with egg wash.

6. Open air fryer, place empanadas in a single layer into heated fryer basket, then shut with lid, cook for 10 minutes, then flip the empanadas and continue cooking for 5 to 7 minutes or until cooked through.
7. Serve straightaway.

Herb Crusted Pork Chops

Servings: 4

Total time: 17 minutes

Nutrition Value:

Calories: 234.7 Cal, Carbs: 1.9 g, Fat: 10.3 g, Protein: 31.9 g, Fiber: 0.5 g.

Smart Points Per Serving: 1

Ingredients:

- 1-pound pork loin chops
- 1 tablespoon herb and garlic seasoning
- 1 teaspoon olive oil

Method:

1. Switch on the air fryer, then insert fryer basket greased with non-stick cooking spray, shut with its lid and preheat at 350 degrees F for 5 minutes.
2. Meanwhile, coat pork chops with oil and then season with herb and garlic seasoning.
3. Open air fryer, place pork chops into heated fryer basket, then shut with lid and cook at 325 degrees F for 12 minutes, flipping chops halfway through.
4. When done, transfer pork chops to a cutting board, let rest for 10 minutes and then serve.

Pork Taquitos

Servings: 5
Total time: 20 minutes

Nutrition Value:

Calories: 256 Cal, Carbs: 23.4 g, Fat: 4 g, Protein: 31.2 g, Fiber: 4 g.

Smart Points Per Serving: 8

Ingredients:

- 30-ounce shredded pork tenderloin, cooked
- 2 1/2 cups grated mozzarella cheese
- 10 small flour tortillas
- 1 lime, juiced
- Salsa for dipping

Method:

1. Switch on the air fryer, then insert heat fryer pan greased with non-stick cooking spray, shut with its lid and preheat at 380 degrees F for 10 minutes.
2. Meanwhile, place pork in a bowl, drizzle with lime juice and stir until mixed.
3. Place tortillas in a heatproof plate, cover with a damp paper towel and microwave for 10 to 20 seconds or until heated through.
4. Working on one tortilla at a time, spread 3-ounce pork on it, then top with ¼ cup cheese and roll it up tightly.
5. Open air fryer, line rolls into heated air fryer pan, spray with oil, then shut with lid and cook for 7 to 10 minutes or until nicely golden brown.
6. When air fryer beeps, open the air fryer, transfer tortillas on a serving plate and serve with salsa.

Breaded Pork Chops

Servings: 6

Total time: 34 minutes

Nutrition Value:

Calories: 273.7 Cal, Carbs: 13.9 g, Fat: 12.2 g, Protein: 25.2 g, Fiber: 1 g.

Smart Points Per Serving: 3

Ingredients:

- 6 boneless pork chops, fat trimmed and each about 5-inch thick
- 1/2 teaspoon onion powder
- 1/2 teaspoon garlic powder
- 1 ¼ teaspoon salt
- 1/8 teaspoon ground black pepper
- ¼ teaspoon red chili powder
- 1 ¼ teaspoon sweet paprika
- ½ cup panko crumbs
- 1/3 cup crushed cornflakes crumbs
- 2 tablespoons grated parmesan cheese
- 1 egg, beaten

Method:

1. Switch on the air fryer, then insert fryer basket greased with non-stick cooking spray, shut with its lid and preheat at 400 degrees F for 10 minutes.
2. Meanwhile, place all crumbs in a bowl, season with a ¾ teaspoon salt, onion powder, garlic powder, black pepper, red chili powder, paprika and cheese and stir until mixed.
3. Crack an egg in a bowl and whisk until beaten.
4. Season pork chops with a ½ teaspoon salt, then dip into the egg mixture and dredge with crumb mixture until evenly coated.

5. Open air fryer, place chops in a single layer into heated fryer basket, then shut with lid and cook for 12 minutes, flipping pork chops halfway through.
6. When air fryer beeps, open the air fryer, transfer chops to a plate and cook in the same manner.
7. Serve pork chops straightaway.

Honey Mustard Pork Chops

Servings: 4

Total time: 18 minutes

Nutrition Value:

Calories: 42.4 Cal, Carbs: 2.9 g, Fat: 1.3 g, Protein: 3.9 g, Fiber: 0 g.

Smart Points Per Serving: 1

Ingredients:

- 1-pound boneless pork chops
- 1 teaspoon steak seasoning blend
- 2 teaspoons honey
- 1 tablespoon mustard paste

Method:

1. Switch on the air fryer, then insert fryer basket greased with non-stick cooking spray, shut with its lid and preheat at 350degrees F for 5 minutes.
2. Meanwhile, whisk together seasoning, honey, and mustard until combined and then crush on all sides of pork chops.
3. Open air fryer, place pork chops in a single layer into heated fryer basket, then shut with lid and cook for 12 minutes, flipping pork chops halfway through.
4. Serve straightaway.

Steak

Servings: 2

Total time: 20 minutes

Nutrition Value:

Calories: 470 Cal, Carbs: 0.5 g, Fat: 31 g, Protein: 45 g, Fiber: 0 g.

Smart Points Per Serving: 0

Ingredients:

- 2 medium-sized rib eye steaks
- 1 teaspoon salt
- ½ teaspoon ground black pepper

Method:

1. Switch on the air fryer, then insert fryer basket greased with non-stick cooking spray, shut with its lid and preheat at 400 degrees F for 5 minutes.
2. Meanwhile, season steaks with salt and black pepper.
3. Open air fryer, place steaks into heated fryer basket, then shut with lid and cook for 14 minutes or until cooked to desired doneness, flipping steaks halfway through.
4. When done, wrap steak into aluminum foil and let rest for 5 minutes before serving.

Meatballs

Servings: 8

Total time: 25 minutes

Nutrition Value:

Calories: 226 Cal, Carbs: 2 g, Fat: 12 g, Protein: 27 g, Fiber: 0 g.

Smart Points Per Serving: 5

Ingredients:

- 1-pound ground chicken
- 1 teaspoon minced garlic
- 2 teaspoons grated ginger
- 1/2 teaspoon salt
- 1/2 teaspoon ground black pepper
- 1/4 teaspoon red pepper flakes
- ¼ cup chopped cilantro

Method:

1. Switch on the air fryer, then insert fryer basket greased with non-stick cooking spray, shut with its lid and preheat at 400 degrees F for 5 minutes.
2. Meanwhile, place all the ingredients in a bowl, stir well until combined and then shape mixture into 16 meatballs.
3. Open air fryer, place meatballs in a single layer into heated fryer basket, then shut with lid and cook at 400 degrees F for 10 minutes, turning meatballs halfway through.
4. When air fryer beeps, open the air fryer, transfer meatballs to a plate and cook remaining meatballs in the same manner.
5. Serve straightaway.

Lamb Chops

Servings: 8

Total time: 15 minutes

Nutrition Value:

Calories: 206 Cal, Carbs: 1.5 g, Fat: 8 g, Protein: 29 g, Fiber: 0.5 g.

Smart Points Per Serving: 4

Ingredients:

- 8 lamb loin chops, each about 3.5 ounce
- 1 ½ teaspoon minced garlic
- 1 ¼ teaspoon salt
- ½ teaspoon ground black pepper
- 1 tablespoon Za'atar
- ½ of lemon, juiced
- 1 teaspoon olive oil

Method:

1. Switch on the air fryer, then insert fryer basket greased with non-stick cooking spray, shut with its lid and preheat at 400 degrees F for 5 minutes.
2. Meanwhile, rub chops with oil and garlic, then drizzle with lemon juice and season with salt, black pepper, and Za'atar seasoning.
3. Open air fryer, place lamb chops into heated fryer basket, then shut with lid and cook for 10 minutes, flipping chops halfway through.
4. Serve straightaway..

Chapter7: Poultry

Chicken Parmesan

Servings: 8
Total time: 30 minutes

Nutrition Value:

Calories: 251 Cal, Carbs: 14 g, Fat: 9.5 g, Protein: 31.5 g, Fiber: 1.5 g.

Smart Points Per Serving: 4

Ingredients:

- 2 chicken breasts, each about 8 ounces and halved
- 6 tablespoons seasoned breadcrumbs
- 1 tablespoon olive oil
- 2 tablespoons grated Parmesan cheese
- 6 tablespoons grated mozzarella cheese
- 1/2 cup marinara sauce

Method:

1. Switch on the air fryer, then insert fryer basket greased with non-stick cooking spray, shut with its lid and preheat at 360 degrees F for 9 minutes.
2. Meanwhile, stir together breadcrumbs and cheese in a shallow dish.
3. Brush oil on all over the chicken and then coat with breadcrumbs mixture.
4. Open air fryer, place breaded chicken in a single layer into heated fryer basket, then shut with lid and cook for 6 minutes.
5. Then turn the chicken, spread with 1 tablespoon of marinara sauce, sprinkle with 1 ½ tablespoon mozzarella cheese and continue air frying for 3 minutes or until cheese melts.
6. Cook remaining chicken in the same manner and serve straightaway.

Buffalo Chicken Taquitos

Servings: 12
Total time: 45 minutes

Nutrition Value:

Calories: 148 Cal, Carbs: 8.32 g, Fat: 8 g, Protein: 13.65 g, Fiber: 4 g.

Smart Points Per Serving: 3

Ingredients:

- 2 cups cooked and shredded chicken breast
- 2 tablespoons buffalo sauce
- 8-ounce cream cheese, low-fat
- 12 small sized flour tortillas, low-carb
- Ranch Dressing as needed

Method:

1. Switch on the air fryer, then insert fryer basket greased with non-stick cooking spray, shut with its lid and preheat at 400 degrees F for 10 minutes.
2. Meanwhile, whisk together buffalo sauce and cream cheese until smooth, then add chicken and stir until combined.
3. Prepare taquitos and for this, place tortillas on a clean working space, spread with chicken buffalo mixture, about 3 tablespoons onto the center and roll.
4. Open air fryer, place taquitos in a single layer into heated fryer basket, spray with oil then shut with lid and cook for 16 minutes or until nicely golden brown.
5. Air fry remaining taquitos in the same manner and serve.

Feta Stuffed Chicken

Servings: 4

Total time: 30 minutes

Nutrition Value:

Calories: 248.8 Cal, Carbs: 20.4 g, Fat: 5.7 g, Protein: 28.3 g, Fiber: 1 g.

Smart Points Per Serving: 2

Ingredients:

- 4 skinless chicken breast halves
- 1/8 teaspoon ground black pepper
- ½ teaspoon dried basil
- 2 teaspoons olive oil
- 1 tablespoon Spaghetti sauce
- 1/4 cup crumbled feta cheese
- 2 tablespoons cream cheese, fat-free
- Salad greens for serving

Method:

1. Switch on the air fryer, then insert fryer basket greased with non-stick cooking spray, shut with its lid and preheat at 370 degrees F for 10 minutes.
2. Meanwhile, stir together basil, cheeses and spaghetti sauce until combined.
3. Cut chicken breast to create a pocket, then stuff evenly with prepared cheese mixture and sprinkle with black pepper.
4. Open air fryer, place stuffed chicken in a single layer into heated fryer basket, then shut with lid and cook for 20 minutes, shaking the basket halfway through.
5. Cook remaining stuffed chicken in the same manner and serve with salad greens.

Chicken Shawarma Salad

Servings: 4

Total time: 20 minutes

Nutrition Value:

Calories: 313 Cal, Carbs: 12 g, Fat: 17 g, Protein: 29 g, Fiber: 3 g.

Smart Points Per Serving: 0

Ingredients:

For the Shawarma:

- 1-pound chicken thighs, cut into bite-sized pieces
- 1 teaspoon salt
- ½ teaspoon allspice
- 2 teaspoons dried oregano
- 1 teaspoon cinnamon
- 1 teaspoon cumin
- 1 teaspoon coriander
- 2 tablespoons olive oil

For The Salad:

- 1 ½ cup cherry tomatoes, halved
- 1 cup cauliflower rice, cooked
- 1 small cucumber, sliced
- 2 cups mixed salad greens
- 1 cup pitted olives

Method:

1. Switch on the air fryer, then insert fryer basket greased with non-stick cooking spray, shut with its lid and preheat at 350 degrees F for 5 minutes.

2. Meanwhile, place all the ingredients for shawarma except for chicken in a shallow dish and whisk until combined, then add chicken and turn until evenly coated.
3. Open air fryer, place chicken into heated fryer basket, then shut with lid and cook for 15 minutes, shaking the basket halfway through.
4. In the meantime, layer salad bowls evenly with tomatoes, cauliflower rice, cucumber, salad greens, and olives.
5. When air fryer beeps, open the air fryer, distribute chicken into salad bowls and serve.

Turkey Breast

Servings: 3

Total time: 30 minutes

Nutrition Value:

Calories: 153 Cal, Carbs: 0 g, Fat: 0.8 g, Protein: 34 g, Fiber: 0 g.

Smart Points Per Serving: 0

Ingredients:

- 1 turkey breast tenderloin
- ½ teaspoon pink salt
- ½ teaspoon ground black pepper
- ½ teaspoon paprika
- ½ teaspoon sage
- ½ teaspoon dried thyme

Method:

1. Switch on the air fryer, then insert fryer basket greased with non-stick cooking spray, shut with its lid and preheat at 350 degrees F for 5 minutes.
2. Meanwhile, stir together salt, black pepper, paprika, sage, and thyme and then rub this mixture all over turkey.
3. Open air fryer, place the seasoned turkey into heated fryer basket, spray with oil, then shut with lid and cook for 25 minutes, flipping turkey halfway through.
4. Serve straightaway.

Chicken Nuggets

Servings: 8

Total time: 20 minutes

Nutrition Value:

Calories: 188 Cal, Carbs: 8 g, Fat: 4.5 g, Protein: 25 g, Fiber: 0 g.

Smart Points Per Serving: 3

Ingredients:

- 6 oz boneless chicken breasts, cut into 1-inch pieces
- ½ teaspoon salt
- ½ teaspoon ground black pepper
- 6 tablespoons Italian breadcrumbs
- 2 tablespoons panko breadcrumbs
- 2 teaspoons olive oil
- 2 tablespoons grated parmesan cheese

Method:

1. Switch on the air fryer, then insert fryer basket greased with non-stick cooking spray, shut with its lid and preheat at 400 degrees F for 10 minutes.
2. Meanwhile, place oil in one shallow dish and place all breadcrumbs in another shallow dish, add cheese and stir until mixed.
3. Season chicken with salt and black pepper, then coat with olive oil and dredge with crumbs mixture.
4. Open air fryer, place breaded chicken breasts into heated fryer basket, then shut with lid and cook for 8 minutes until nicely golden brown, turning chicken halfway through.
5. Serve straightaway.

Cheesy Ranch Chicken

Servings: 4

Total time: 26 minutes

Nutrition Value:

Calories: 279 Cal, Carbs: 11 g, Fat: 8 g, Protein: 36 g, Fiber: 0 g.

Smart Points Per Serving: 3

Ingredients:

- 1.25 pounds skinless chicken tenderloins
- ½ teaspoon salt
- 1/8 teaspoon ground black pepper
- ½ teaspoon dried parsley
- ½ teaspoon paprika
- ½ cup corn flake crumbs
- ½ cup Ranch Greek Yogurt Dip
- 2 tablespoons grated cheddar cheese

Method:

1. Switch on the air fryer, then insert fryer basket greased with non-stick cooking spray, shut with its lid and preheat at 350 degrees F for 10 minutes.
2. Meanwhile, place yogurt in a bowl, add cheese and whisk until combined.
3. Place crumbs in a shallow dish, add salt, black pepper, paprika, parsley, and crumbs and stir until combined.
4. Brush chicken with yogurt mixture until evenly coated on all side, then dredge with crumbs mixture.
5. Open air fryer, place chicken in a single layer into heated fryer basket, then shut with lid and cook for 16 minutes, turning chicken halfway through.
6. Serve straightaway.

Whole Roasted Chicken

Servings: 8

Total time: 1 hour and 25 minutes

Nutrition Value:

Calories: 263.4 Cal, Carbs: 28.6 g, Fat: 6 g, Protein: 23.5 g, Fiber: 4.8 g.

Smart Points Per Serving: 3

Ingredients:

- 5 Pound Chicken
- 1 cup cauliflower florets
- 2 cups broccoli florets
- 2 cups baby carrots
- 2 teaspoons Salt
- 1 teaspoon ground black Pepper
- 4 tablespoons lemon pepper seasoning
- 1 Lemon, quartered
- 1 lime, halved
- ¼ cup chopped cilantro
- 3 tablespoons olive oil

Method:

1. Switch on the air fryer, then insert fryer basket greased with non-stick cooking spray, shut with its lid and preheat at 380 degrees F for 10 minutes.
2. Meanwhile, coat chicken with oil, then sprinkle lemon pepper seasoning over and under the skin of the chicken and stuff with lemon pieces.
3. Open air fryer, place chicken in upside down position into heated fryer basket, then shut with lid and cook for 1 hour, turning chicken halfway through.

4. In the meantime, place a large pot half full with water over medium-high heat, bring the water to boil, then add cauliflower, broccoli and carrots in it and broil for 3 to 4 minutes.
5. Then drain vegetables, sprinkle with salt and black pepper and spray with oil.
6. When air fryer beeps, open the air fryer, transfer chicken to a cutting board and wrap in aluminum foil.
7. Add seasoned vegetables into the air fryer, shut with lid and cook for 15 minutes at 400 degrees F, shaking vegetables halfway through.
8. When done, garnish vegetables with cilantro and serve with lime and chicken.

Chapter 8: Vegetarian

Tofu

Servings: 4
Total time: 17 minutes

Nutrition Value:

Calories: 63 Cal, Carbs: 4 g, Fat: 1 g, Protein: 7 g, Fiber: 1 g.

Smart Points Per Serving: 0

Ingredients:

- 14 ounces extra-firm tofu
- ½ teaspoon sea salt
- 1 teaspoon smoked paprika
- 1/2 teaspoon ground coriander
- 1 tablespoon cornstarch

Method:

1. Switch on the air fryer, then insert fryer basket greased with non-stick cooking spray, shut with its lid and preheat at 375 degrees F for 5 minutes.
2. Meanwhile, stir together salt, paprika, coriander, and cornstarch until combined and then add to a resealable plastic bag.
3. Cut tofu into bite-size pieces, seal the bag and turn it upside down until tofu is evenly coated with spices.
4. Open air fryer, place tofu in a single layer into heated fryer basket, then shut with lid and cook for 12 minutes, turning halfway through.
5. Serve straightaway.

Vegetable Kebab

Servings: 3

Total time: 20 minutes

Nutrition Value:

Calories: 81 Cal, Carbs: 17 g, Fat: 1 g, Protein: 3 g, Fiber: 7 g.

Smart Points Per Serving: 0

Ingredients:

- 2 medium green bell peppers, cored
- 1 medium eggplant, destemmed
- 1 medium zucchini, ends trimmed
- ½ of white onion, peeled
- 1 teaspoon salt
- ½ teaspoon ground black pepper
- Wooden skewers as needed

Method:

1. Switch on the air fryer, then insert fryer basket greased with non-stick cooking spray, shut with its lid and preheat at 390 degrees F for 10 minutes.
2. Meanwhile, place skewers in a bowl, pour in warm water to cover them and set aside.
3. Cut peppers, eggplant, zucchini, and onion into 1-inch cubes, then thread vegetables into soaked skewers, spray with oil and season with salt and black pepper.
4. Open air fryer, place vegetable skewers in a single layer into heated fryer basket, then shut with lid and cook at 390 degrees F for 10 minutes, turning halfway through.
5. Serve straightaway.

Baked Potatoes

Servings: 2

Total time: 45 minutes

Nutrition Value:

Calories: 161 Cal, Carbs: 37 g, Fat: 0.2 g, Protein: 4.3 g, Fiber: 3.8 g.

Smart Points Per Serving: 1

Ingredients:

- 2 medium potatoes
- 1 tablespoon chopped parsley
- 2 tablespoons unsalted butter

Method:

1. Switch on the air fryer, then insert fryer basket greased with non-stick cooking spray, shut with its lid and preheat at 400 degrees F for 5 minutes.
2. Meanwhile, use a fork to prick potatoes and then spray with oil.
3. Open air fryer, place potatoes into heated fryer basket, then shut with lid and cook for 30 to 40 minutes or until tender, turning potatoes halfway through.
4. When done, slice the potatoes down to the center and top with butter.
5. Sprinkle potatoes with parsley and serve.

Savory Squash Wedges

Servings: 4

Total time: 18 minutes;

Nutrition Value:

Calories: 66.9 Cal, Carbs: 14.9 g, Fat: 1.3 g, Protein: 1.3 g, Fiber: 4.2 g.

Smart Points Per Serving: 0

Ingredients:

- 1 medium butternut squash
- 2 tablespoons nutritional yeast
- 2 tablespoons dipping seasoning

Method:

1. Switch on the air fryer, then insert fryer basket greased with non-stick cooking spray, shut with its lid and preheat at 400 degrees F for 10 minutes.
2. Meanwhile, cut the squash into half, then remove its seeds, cut its flesh into crescent shape slices.
3. Spray butternut squash pieces with oil and season with yeast and dipping seasoning.
4. Open air fryer, place seasoned squash pieces in a single layer into heated fryer basket, then shut with lid and cook for 8 minutes, shaking the basket halfway through.
5. Serve straightaway.

Cajun Zucchini Chips

Servings: 2

Total time: 32 minutes

Nutrition Value:

Calories: 63.9 Cal, Carbs: 8.2 g, Fat: 2 g, Protein: 4 g, Fiber: 1.7 g.

Smart Points Per Serving: 0

Ingredients:

- 1 medium zucchini
- 1 teaspoon Cajun seasoning

Method:

1. Switch on the air fryer, then insert fryer basket greased with non-stick cooking spray, shut with its lid and preheat at 370 degrees F for 8 minutes.
2. Meanwhile, cut zucchini into 1/8-inch slices, then spray with oil and season with Cajun seasoning until evenly coated on all sides.
3. Open air fryer, place seasoned zucchini slices in a single layer into heated fryer basket, then shut with lid and cook for 16 minutes, flipping zucchini slices halfway through.
4. Serve straightaway.

Buffalo Cauliflower Wings

Servings: 4

Total time: 32 minutes

Nutrition Value:

Calories: 66 Cal, Carbs: 1 g, Fat: 4 g, Protein: 6 g, Fiber: 2 g.

Smart Points Per Serving: 1

Ingredients:

- 1 medium head of cauliflower, cut into florets
- 1 tablespoon almond flour
- ½ teaspoon salt
- 1 tablespoon avocado oil
- 4 tablespoons hot sauce

Method:

1. Switch on the air fryer, then insert fryer basket greased with non-stick cooking spray, shut with its lid and preheat at 400 degrees F for 5 minutes.
2. Meanwhile, whisk together flour, salt, oil and hot sauce in a shallow dish, then add cauliflower florets and stir until well coated.
3. Open air fryer, place cauliflower florets in a single layer into heated fryer basket, then shut with lid and cook for 15 minutes, shaking the basket halfway through.
4. When air fryer beeps, open the air fryer, transfer fried cauliflower florets in a dish, then add remaining cauliflower florets into the air fryer and cook for 12 minutes.
5. Serve straightaway.

Brussels Sprouts

Servings: 4

Total time: 20 minutes

Nutrition Value:

Calories: 135 Cal, Carbs: 11 g, Fat: 9.8 g, Protein: 3.9 g, Fiber: 4 g.

Smart Points Per Serving: 0

Ingredients:

- 1-pound Brussels sprouts, halved
- 1 teaspoon salt
- ½ teaspoon ground black pepper
- 2 tablespoons olive oil

Method:

1. Switch on the air fryer, then insert fryer basket greased with non-stick cooking spray, shut with its lid and preheat at 350 degrees F for 5 minutes.
2. Meanwhile, place sprouts in a large bowl, season with salt and black pepper, drizzle with oil and toss until well coated.
3. Open air fryer, place sprouts into heated fryer basket, then shut with lid and cook for 12 minutes, shaking the basket halfway through.
4. Serve straightaway.

Green Beans

Servings: 4

Total time: 20 minutes

Nutrition Value:

Calories: 44 Cal, Carbs: 10 g, Fat: 0 g, Protein: 2 g, Fiber: 4 g.

Smart Points Per Serving: 0

Ingredients:

- 1-pound green beans
- 1 teaspoon salt
- 2 tablespoons olive oil

Method:

1. Switch on the air fryer, then insert fryer basket greased with non-stick cooking spray, shut with its lid and preheat at 400 degrees F for 10 minutes.
2. Meanwhile, place green beans in a shallow dish, season with salt, add oil and toss until well coated.
3. Open air fryer, place beans into heated fryer basket, then shut with lid and cook at 325 degrees F for 8 minutes, shaking the basket halfway through.
4. Serve straightaway.

Chapter 9: Fish and Seafood

Salt and Pepper Shrimp

Servings: 2
Total time: 20 minutes

Nutrition Value:

Calories: 56 Cal, Carbs: 3.2 g, Fat: 1.7 g, Protein: 6.6 g, Fiber: 0.2 g.

Smart Points Per Serving: 0

Ingredients:

- 8-ounce shrimps, peeled and deveined
- ¼ teaspoon sea salt
- ¼ and 1/8 teaspoon sugar
- ¼ and 1/8 teaspoon ground white pepper
- 1 1/2 teaspoons cornstarch
- 1 ½ teaspoon olive oil

Method:

1. Switch on the air fryer, then insert fryer basket greased with non-stick cooking spray, shut with its lid and preheat at 450 degrees F for 5 minutes.
2. Meanwhile, place salt, sugar, white pepper and cornstarch in a shallow dish, stir until mixed, then add shrimp and toss until well coated.
3. Then drizzle 1 ½ teaspoon oil over shrimps and toss until coated.
4. Open air fryer, place shrimps in a single layer into heated fryer basket, then shut with lid and cook for 2 minutes or until top side is crispy, then turn shrimps and cook for another 1 ½ minute.
5. Serve straightaway.

Tuna Cakes

Servings: 4

Total time: 20 minutes

Nutrition Value:

Calories: 116.4 Cal, Carbs: 9.8 g, Fat: 2.2 g, Protein: 13.6 g, Fiber: 1 g.

Smart Points Per Serving: 1

Ingredients:

- 3-ounce cooked tuna
- 1 tablespoon flour
- ⅛ teaspoon garlic powder
- ⅛ teaspoon salt
- ⅛ teaspoon ground black pepper
- ⅛ teaspoon dried dill
- 1 teaspoon mayonnaise

Method:

1. Switch on the air fryer, then insert fryer basket greased with non-stick cooking spray, shut with its lid and preheat at 380 degrees F for 10 minutes.
2. Meanwhile, place tuna in a bowl, then add remaining ingredients, stir until combined and then shape mixture into 4 patties.
3. Open air fryer, place patties into heated fryer basket, spray with oil, then shut with lid and cook for 10 minutes, turning patties halfway through.
4. Serve straightaway.

Coconut Shrimp

Servings: 4

Total time: 20 minutes

Nutrition Value:

Calories: 63 Cal, Carbs: 6 g, Fat: 3.3 g, Protein: 2.2 g, Fiber: 0.4 g.

Smart Points Per Serving: 4

Ingredients:

- 16-ounce large shrimp, peeled and deveined
- ½ teaspoon salt
- ¼ teaspoon cayenne pepper
- ½ cup panko breadcrumbs
- ½ cup shredded coconut, unsweetened
- 2 egg whites

Method:

1. Switch on the air fryer, then insert fryer basket greased with non-stick cooking spray, shut with its lid and preheat at 400 degrees F for 10 minutes.
2. Meanwhile, place salt, pepper, breadcrumbs, and coconut in a shallow dish and stir until mixed.
3. Place eggs in a bowl and whisk until blended, then dip shrimp into the egg mixture and dredge into breadcrumbs mixture until evenly coated.
4. Open air fryer, place shrimp in a single layer into heated fryer basket, then shut with lid and cook for 5 minutes, shaking the basket halfway through.
5. Cook remaining shrimps in the same manner and serve.

Ranch Fish Fillets

Servings: 2

Total time: 20 minutes

Nutrition Value:

Calories: 239 Cal, Carbs: 16.6 g, Fat: 2 g, Protein: 35.2 g, Fiber: 0 g.

Smart Points Per Serving: 2

Ingredients:

- 4 tilapia salmon
- ¾ cup crushed cornflakes
- 2 tablespoons ranch seasoning
- 2 ½ tablespoons olive oil
- 2 eggs, beaten

Method:

1. Switch on the air fryer, then insert fryer basket greased with non-stick cooking spray, shut with its lid and preheat at 350 degrees F for 10 minutes.
2. Meanwhile, place cornflakes and ranch seasoning in a shallow dish and stir until combined.
3. Crack eggs in a bowl, whisk until beaten, then dip salmon in it and dredge into cornflakes mixture until evenly coated
4. Open air fryer, place salmon into heated fryer basket, spray with oil, then shut with lid and cook for 12 minutes, turning salmon halfway through.
5. Serve straightaway.

Fried Cat Fish

Servings: 4

Total time: 30 minutes

Nutrition Value:

Calories: 182 Cal, Carbs: 5 g, Fat: 12.8 g, Protein: 11.12 g, Fiber: 0.2 g.

Smart Points Per Serving: 0

Ingredients:

- 4 fillets of catfish
- ¼ cup fish fry seasoning
- 1 tablespoon chopped parsley
- 1 tablespoon olive oil

Method:

1. Switch on the air fryer, then insert fryer basket greased with non-stick cooking spray, shut with its lid and preheat at 400 degrees F for 10 minutes.
2. Meanwhile, place seasoning in a large resealable plastic bag, add fillets, then seal the bag and turn it upside down until fillet is well coated with the seasoning.
3. Open air fryer, place seasoned fillets into heated fryer basket, spray with oil, then shut with lid and cook at 400 degrees F for 20 minutes or until nicely golden brown and crispy, flipping fish fillet halfway through.
4. Garnish with parsley and serve straightaway.

Sriracha Salmon

Servings: 4

Total time: 30 minutes

Nutrition Value:

Calories: 196 Cal, Carbs: 4 g, Fat: 8.9 g, Protein: 24.6 g, Fiber: 0.2 g.

Smart Points Per Serving: 2

Ingredients:

- 4 salmon fillets, each about 5 ounces
- 1 ½ tablespoon minced garlic
- 1 teaspoon salt
- ½ teaspoon ground black pepper
- 3 tablespoons honey
- 1 ½ teaspoon Sriracha sauce
- 2 tablespoons Worcestershire sauce
- 4 tablespoons unsalted butter, softened
- 1 lime, juiced

Method:

1. Switch on the air fryer, then insert fryer basket greased with non-stick cooking spray, shut with its lid and preheat at 370 degrees F for 10 minutes.
2. Meanwhile, place all the ingredients except for salmon in a shallow dish and whisk until combined.
3. Then add salmon fillets and turn into the sauce until well coated.
4. Open air fryer, place salmon fillets in a single layer into heated fryer basket, then shut with lid and cook for 10 minutes, turning salmon halfway through.
5. Cook remaining salmon fillets in the same manner and serve.

Fish Sticks

Servings: 8
Total time: 26 minutes

Nutrition Value:

Calories: 250 Cal, Carbs: 24 g, Fat: 11 g, Protein: 14 g, Fiber: 2 g.

Smart Points Per Serving: 6

Ingredients:

- 1-pound tilapia fillets
- 1 ½ cups Fiber One Cereal
- ½ cup whole wheat flour
- 1 teaspoon garlic powder
- 1 teaspoon salt
- ½ teaspoon ground black pepper
- 1 teaspoon lemon pepper seasoning
- ½ teaspoon paprika
- ½ cup egg substitute

Method:

1. Switch on the air fryer, then insert fryer basket greased with non-stick cooking spray, shut with its lid and preheat at 400 degrees F for 10 minutes.
2. Meanwhile, place cereal in a food processor, add garlic, salt, paprika and lemon pepper seasoning and pulse for 1 minute or until finely ground, transfer in a shallow dish.
3. Place flour in another shallow dish and egg substitute in another dish.
4. Cut fillet into 3-inch strips, then coat each fillet with flour, dip into egg and dredge with breadcrumbs.

5. Open air fryer, place coated fillets in a single layer into heated fryer basket, then shut with lid and cook for 8 minutes or until nicely golden brown, turning fillets halfway through.
6. Cook remaining fillets in the same manner and serve.

Cilantro Lime Shrimp Skewers

Servings: 4

Total time: 26 minutes

Nutrition Value:

Calories: 59 Cal, Carbs: 2 g, Fat: 1 g, Protein: 11 g, Fiber: 0 g.

Smart Points Per Serving: 0

Ingredients:

- ½ pound raw shrimp, peeled and deveined
- ½ teaspoon minced garlic
- ¾ teaspoon salt
- ½ teaspoon paprika
- ½ teaspoon ground cumin
- 1 tablespoon chopped cilantro
- 1 lemon, juiced

Method:

1. Switch on the air fryer, then insert fryer basket greased with non-stick cooking spray, shut with its lid and preheat at 350 degrees F for 10 minutes.
2. Meanwhile, place all the ingredients except for shrimps and cilantro in a shallow dish and stir until mixed.
3. Then add shrimps into the spice mixture, toss until evenly coated and thread onto skewers.
4. Open air fryer, place shrimp skewers in a single layer into heated fryer basket, spray with oil, then shut with lid and cook for 8 minutes, turning shrimps halfway through.
5. Cook remaining shrimp skewers in the same manner and serve.

Salmon

Servings: 2

Total time: 20 minutes

Nutrition Value:

Calories: 161 Cal, Carbs: 2 g, Fat: 7 g, Protein: 22 g, Fiber: 2 g.

Smart Points Per Serving: 0

Ingredients:

- 2 fillets of salmon
- ½ teaspoon salt
- ½ teaspoon paprika
- 1/8 teaspoon ground cardamom

Method:

1. Switch on the air fryer, then insert fryer basket greased with non-stick cooking spray, shut with its lid and preheat at 350 degrees F for 10 minutes.
2. Meanwhile, spray fillets with oil, season with salt and black pepper and sprinkle with paprika and cardamom.
3. Open air fryer, place fillets into heated fryer basket, then shut with lid and cook for 12 minutes, turning fillet halfway through.
4. Serve straightaway.

Salmon Patties

Servings: 18

Total time: 20 minutes

Nutrition Value:

Calories: 118.5 Cal, Carbs: 5 g, Fat: 4.8 g, Protein: 15.8 g, Fiber: 0.1 g.

Smart Points Per Serving: 0

Ingredients:

- 14 ounces cooked salmon
- 3 tablespoons chopped cilantro
- 3 green onions, minced
- ½ teaspoon salt
- 1 teaspoon smoked paprika
- 1 egg

Method:

1. Switch on the air fryer, then insert fryer basket greased with non-stick cooking spray, shut with its lid and preheat at 360 degrees F for 10 minutes.
2. Meanwhile, place salmon in a bowl, mince it with a hand, then add remaining ingredients, stir until combined and then shape mixture into 6 patties.
3. Open air fryer, place patties in a single layer into heated fryer basket, spray with oil, then shut with lid and cook for 8 minutes, turning patties halfway through.
4. Serve straightaway.

Chapter 10: Desserts

Pop Tarts

Servings: 6
Total time: 20 minutes

Nutrition Value:

Calories: 200 Cal, Carbs: 38 g, Fat: 5 g, Protein: 2 g, Fiber: 0.5 g.

Smart Points Per Serving: 2

Ingredients:

- 1 cup self-rising flour
- Raspberry preserves as needed, sugar-free
- 1/4 cup powdered sugar
- 1 cup Greek yogurt, nonfat

Method:

1. Switch on the air fryer, then insert fryer basket greased with non-stick cooking spray, shut with its lid and preheat at 325 degrees F for 10 minutes.
2. Meanwhile, place flour in a bowl, add yogurt and stir well until combined.
3. Transfer dough to a clean working space, knead until a smooth dough comes together, then roll it out and cut into twelve rectangles.
4. Spread raspberry preserves on top of six rectangles, leaving a ¼ inch of rectangle, then cover with other rectangle and seal with a fork.
5. Open air fryer, place tarts in a single layer into heated fryer basket, then shut with lid and cook for 10 minutes.
6. Cook remaining tarts in the same manner, then sprinkle with powdered sugar and serve.

Apple Chips with Cinnamon

Servings: 6

Total time: 28 minutes

Nutrition Value:

Calories: 117 Cal, Carbs: 31.9 g, Fat: 0.9 g, Protein: 0.8 g, Fiber: 11.1 g.

Smart Points Per Serving: 0

Ingredients:

- 3 large sweet apples, unpeeled
- ¾ teaspoons cinnamon
- 1/8 teaspoon salt

Method:

1. Switch on the air fryer, then insert fryer basket greased with non-stick cooking spray, shut with its lid and preheat at 390 degrees F for 10 minutes.
2. Meanwhile, rinse apples, remove their core and cut into 1/8-inch round slices.
3. Arrange apple slices in a single layer on a baking sheet, then mix salt and cinnamon and rub this mixture on apple slices.
4. Open air fryer, add apple slices in a single layer into heated fryer basket, then shut with lid and cook for 16 minutes, flipping chips halfway through.
5. Cook remaining chips in the same manner and serve straightaway.

Lemon Muffins

Servings: 8

Total time: 24 minutes

Nutrition Value:

Calories: 314 Cal, Carbs: 28 g, Fat: 18 g, Protein: 10 g, Fiber: 1 g.

Smart Points Per Serving: 2

Ingredients:

- 16-ounce lemon cake mix
- 5.3-ounce lemon flavored Greek yogurt, about 100 calories
- 1 cup water

Method:

1. Switch on the air fryer, then insert fryer basket, shut with its lid and preheat at 320 degrees F for 10 minutes.
2. Meanwhile, place all the ingredients in a large bowl and stir until smooth batter comes together.
3. Grease silicone muffin tins with oil and then evenly distribute muffin batter in them.
4. Open air fryer, place muffin tins in a single layer into heated fryer basket, then shut with lid and cook for 14 minutes or until muffins are cooked through.
5. Serve straightaway.

Pumpkin Spiced Cookies

Servings: 8

Total time: 30 minutes

Nutrition Value:

Calories: 51 Cal, Carbs: 9.5 g, Fat: 1 g, Protein: 1 g, Fiber: 1 g.

Smart Points Per Serving: 3

Ingredients:

- 1 3/4 cups flour
- ½ teaspoon baking soda
- 1 tablespoon pumpkin spice
- 1 cup and 3 tablespoons sugar, divided
- 1 tablespoon honey
- 1 teaspoon vanilla extract, unsweetened
- ½ teaspoon cream of tartar
- ¼ cup unsalted butter, softened
- 1 egg

Method:

1. Switch on the air fryer, shut with its lid and preheat at 320 degrees F for 15 minutes.
2. Meanwhile, place flour in a bowl, add baking soda and cream of tartar and whisk until combined.
3. Place butter in another bowl, add 1 cup sugar and whisk until well blended and creamy.
4. Beat in honey, vanilla, and egg until combined and then gradually beat in flour mixture until incorporated.
5. Cover the bowl and then place it into the refrigerator for 10 minutes or until chill.
6. Then shape dough into 1-inch balls, about 42.

7. Stir together remaining sugar and pumpkin spice in a shallow dish, roll each cookie ball in it and place in a fryer proof baking pan lined with parchment sheet.
8. Open air fryer, insert pan containing cookies in it, then shut with lid and cook for 7 minutes.
9. When air fryer beeps, open the air fryer, transfer cookies to wire rack and cool completely.
10. Cook remaining cookies, in the same manner, cool completely on a wire rack and serve.

Carrot Cake

Servings: 8

Total time: 25 minutes

Nutrition Value:

Calories: 200 Cal, Carbs: 22 g, Fat: 12 g, Protein: 0 g, Fiber: 0 g.

Smart Points Per Serving: 1.5

Ingredients:

- 15-ounce carrot cake mix
- 5.3-ounce vanilla flavored Greek yogurt, about 100 calories
- 1 cup water

Method:

1. Switch on the air fryer, then insert fryer basket, shut with its lid and preheat at 320 degrees F for 10 minutes.
2. Meanwhile, place all the ingredients for the cake in a large bowl and stir until smooth batter comes together.
3. Grease silicone muffin tins with oil and then evenly distribute muffin batter in them.
4. Open air fryer, place muffin tins in a single layer into heated fryer basket, then shut with lid and cook for 14 minutes or until muffins are cooked through.
5. Serve straightaway.

Funnel Cake Bites

Servings: 32

Total time: 18 minutes

Nutrition Value:

Calories: 276 Cal, Carbs: 29 g, Fat: 14.3 g, Protein: 7.3 g, Fiber: 0.9 g.

Smart Points Per Serving: 3

Ingredients:

- 1 cup self-rising flour, divided
- 1 tablespoon vanilla beans paste
- 1 cup Greek yogurt, nonfat
- Powdered sugar for dusting

Method:

1. Switch on the air fryer, then insert fryer basket greased with non-stick cooking spray, shut with its lid and preheat at 375 degrees F for 10 minutes.
2. Meanwhile, place ¾ cup flour in a bowl, add yogurt and vanilla beans paste and stir until well mixed.
3. Transfer dough to a clean working space, sprinkle with remaining flour, then sprinkle with remaining flour, roll into crust and cut into 32 squares.
4. Open air fryer, place cake squares in a single layer into heated fryer basket, then shut with lid and cook for 8 minutes, flipping cake bites halfway through.
5. Cook remaining cake bites in the same manner, then dust with powdered sugar and serve.

Donuts

Servings: 5

Total time: 18 minutes

Nutrition Value:

Calories: 165 Cal, Carbs: 24 g, Fat: 5 g, Protein: 3 g, Fiber: 0 g.

Smart Points Per Serving: 3

Ingredients:

- 1 cup self-rising flour, divided
- ½ cup cinnamon Splenda mixture
- 1 tablespoon vanilla bean paste
- 1 cup Greek yogurt, nonfat

Method:

1. Switch on the air fryer, then insert fryer basket greased with non-stick cooking spray, shut with its lid and preheat at 375 degrees F for 10 minutes.
2. Meanwhile, place ¾ cup flour in a bowl, add Splenda mixture and vanilla bean paste and stir well until a smooth dough comes together.
3. Transfer dough to a clean surface, sprinkle with remaining dough, then roll into crust.
4. Divide crust into 5 parts and roll each part to make donuts.
5. Open air fryer, place donuts in a single layer into heated fryer basket, spray with oil, then shut with lid and cook for 8 minutes, flipping donuts halfway through.
6. Cook remaining donuts in the same manner and serve.

Cinnamon Rolls

Servings: 8

Total time: 34 minutes

Nutrition Value:

Calories: 290 Cal, Carbs: 47 g, Fat: 9.9 g, Protein: 3.8 g, Fiber: 1.2 g.

Smart Points Per Serving: 1

Ingredients:

- 1 cup self-rising flour
- 1/4 teaspoon vanilla bean paste
- ¾ teaspoon cinnamon, divided
- 1/2 teaspoon Splenda
- 1/2 cup whipped cream cheese
- 2 tablespoons water
- 1 cup Greek yogurt, nonfat

Method:

1. Switch on the air fryer, then insert fryer basket greased with non-stick cooking spray, shut with its lid and preheat at 400 degrees F for 10 minutes.
2. Meanwhile, place flour in a bowl, add ¼ teaspoon cinnamon, vanilla bean pastes and stir until a smooth dough comes together.
3. Transfer dough onto a clean working space, roll into the crust, divide into three pieces and then cut each section into 8 sections.
4. Open air fryer, place rolls in a single layer into heated fryer basket, then shut with lid and cook for 12 minutes, shaking the basket halfway through.
5. Place remaining ingredients in a small bowl and whisk until combined, set aside until required.
6. Cook remaining rolls in the same manner and when done, drizzle with prepared cream cheese mixture and serve.

Conclusion

Maintaining a healthy life along with losing weight by doing less hard work is a very daunting task. If you are looking for something different that can ease your journey to weight loss and healthy life more comfortable and simpler, then you should give Weight Watchers Freestyle a try.

Weight Watchers Freestyle program educates, inspires and motivate you to create your own healthy eating plan, without any limitations. As a result, you will be able to develop and stick to your good eating habits for a long time that will not only help you meet your weight loss target quickly; it will also make your life simpler and more fun than any diets have made it for you.

You will miss your junk food in the beginning, but with time, you won't crave for that stuff anymore. You taste buds and body will adjust itself to eat something good. You will find your success with Weight Watchers this year.

You can do this!

Lightning Source UK Ltd.
Milton Keynes UK
UKHW030639190121
377315UK00009B/817